T0078110

WHAT YOU NEED TO KNOW ABOUT BEAUTIFUL NAILS

A BETTER UNDERSTANDING OF NAIL CHEMISTRY

HARMINDER GILL

authorHOUSE®

AuthorHouse™
1663 Liberty Drive
Bloomington, IN 47403
www.authorhouse.com
Phone: 833-262-8899

© 2020 Harminder Gill. All rights reserved.

No part of this book may be reproduced, stored in a retrieval system, or transmitted by any means without the written permission of the author.

Published by AuthorHouse 09/18/2020

ISBN: 978-1-7283-7139-9 (sc)
ISBN: 978-1-7283-7245-7 (e)

Library of Congress Control Number: 2020916586

Print information available on the last page.

Any people depicted in stock imagery provided by Getty Images are models, and such images are being used for illustrative purposes only. Certain stock imagery © Getty Images.

This book is printed on acid-free paper.

Because of the dynamic nature of the Internet, any web addresses or links contained in this book may have changed since publication and may no longer be valid. The views expressed in this work are solely those of the author and do not necessarily reflect the views of the publisher, and the publisher hereby disclaims any responsibility for them.

Table of Contents

Acknowledgements.............................. vii

Chapter 1   Basic Chemistry 1

Chapter 2   Nail Tips and Wraps..........37

Chapter 3   Nail Enhancements 54

Chapter 4   Different Gels 86

Chapter 5   Nail Products................... 105

References 167

About the Author................................. 171

Acknowledgements

I wish to acknowledge Author House for taking the time to publish this book. Thank you very much for the time and dedication to make this book possible.

Chapter 1

Basic Chemistry

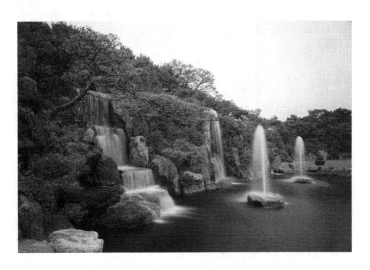

Welcome to the world of the chemistry of nails. It is my pleasure to share some interesting science facts to help those who wear nail polish and any nail products for the nails. Providing nail services is not possible without using chemicals. Everything we can see or touch except both light and electricity is considered to be a chemical. The world we live in, our bodies, and even the numerous gases such as oxygen and nitrogen we breathe are made up of chemicals. Of course, cosmetics is made of chemicals. It is important to understand what chemicals are and how to use them. Nail professionals and even the community needs to have a basic understanding of chemistry.

Chemistry is defined as the science that deals with the composition, structures, and properties of matter and how matter changes during different conditions. Organic chemistry is the study of substances that contain carbon as its element. All living species or even species that were once alive, whether they were plants or animals contain the element carbon. In fact, compounds that contain both carbon and hydrogen are called hydrocarbons and actually react with oxygen gas to produce carbon dioxide and water. We hear the word "organic" as safe or natural because it is associated with living things such as food or food ingredients.

We should be aware that not all organic substances are natural, healthy, or even safe. Gasoline, motor oil, plastics, fabrics, pesticides, and fertilizers are considered to be organic substances. Likewise, all nail enhancements, nail tips, and even nail polishes are considered to be organic chemicals. The bottom line is organic does not mean natural and healthy. It means the substance contains both of the elements carbon and hydrogen from natural or synthetic sources.

Inorganic chemistry is the study of substances that do not contain carbon but might contain hydrogen. Most inorganic substances don't burn because they don't contain carbon and are never considered to be alive. Metals, minerals, glass, water, and air are considered to be inorganic materials or chemicals. For example, the compound titanium dioxide is a white pigment and an inorganic chemical used to whiten polymer powders and Ultra Violet (UV) gels as well as giving opacity in nail polish to provide better coverage.

Matter is any substance that occupies space and has mass. All matter has physical and chemical properties and can exist as either as a solid, liquid, or a gas. All matter is made of chemicals and has the following distinguishing properties such as touch, taste, smell, and vision. This is in contrast to visible light and electricity that we can see but are not made of matter and explains why they are not made of chemicals. Both light and electricity are different forms of energy, and energy is not matter. In fact, everything known to exist in the universe is made up of either matter or energy.

Matter consists of the elements of our world. We can think of elements as the building blocks of nature. Elements are the simplest form of chemical matter and cannot be broken down into simpler substances without losing its identity. Each element has its own distinctive physical and chemical properties. Elements are identified by symbols such as C for carbon, H for hydrogen, O for oxygen, N for nitrogen, S for sulfur, and many other symbols are found on The Periodic Table of Elements.

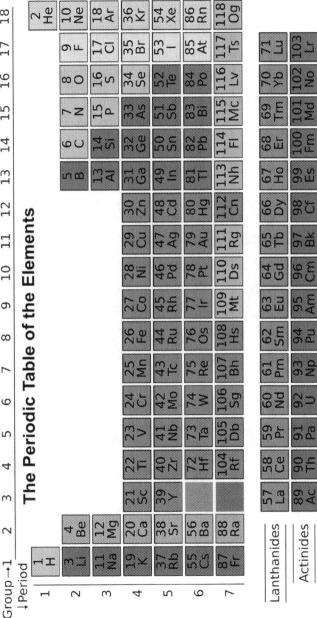

Atoms are the chemicals from which matter is composed, and we can state that matter is made up of entirely of chemicals. Atoms are thought of as the structural units that make up elements. There are different elements that are different from one another because the structure of the atoms are different. Each element is made up of one kind of atom, and it is the differences between atoms that makes one element different from one another. An atom is considered to be the smallest chemical particle for that element and retains the same properties of that element. There is no way that atoms can't be combined into simpler substances by chemical changes.

Molecules are made by combining different atoms which is similar to words being formed by combining different letters of the alphabet. A molecule is thought of as chemical combination of two or more different types of atoms. Water, for example, is made from two atoms of hydrogen and one atom of oxygen. Carbon dioxide is made from one atom of carbon and two atoms of oxygen. Air is mostly composed of nitrogen and oxygen gas. The oxygen we breathe is a molecule that contains two atoms of the element oxygen that are chemically bonded together in fixed proportions. The molecule ozone contains oxygen but three of them chemically combined. Combining atoms of one type of element are called elemental molecules. Compound molecules are made by combining two or more atoms of different elements. For example, sodium chloride is also called table salt and is a chemical compound that contains one atom of the element sodium and one atom of the element chlorine.

The elements and molecules together make up the states of matter. Matter exists in one of three different physical forms such as solid, liquid, or gas depending on its temperature. Water, for example, can exist in three different states of matter, depending on its temperature. When liquid water freezes, it turns solid water which is referred to as ice, and when ice melts, it turns back to liquid water. When liquid water boils, it turns to gaseous water or steam, and when steam cools, it turns back to liquid water. Water is said to undergo physical changes according to changes in temperature, but it still retains the chemical formula and identity H_2O as having two hydrogen atoms for every one oxygen atom. Water can even act as an acid or a base and is referred to as amphoteric.

States of matter have the following distinct characteristics. Solids have a definite shape and volume. Liquids have a definite volume but not a different shape. Gases do not have a definite volume or shape and can't be liquid at normal temperatures and pressures. Plasma can be considered to be a fourth state of matter, but it still behaves like a gas. Unlike gases, plasmas conduct electricity and are found in the Sun and other stars. You will most likely see plasma by observing lightning storms or by looking at neon signs. Electricity is passed through the gases inside the tubes of neon signs where plasma is formed and visible light is emitted.

A vapor is a liquid that has evaporated into the gaseous state, but it is not a gas.

Vapors can return to the liquid state when they cool down enough. Gases have to be highly pressured before they can become liquid, and when the pressure is lowered enough, the liquid can turn into a gas once again. Steam is considered to be vapor. Vapors are not states of matter but liquids that have undergone physical changes.

The physical and chemical changes that these molecules undergo can also be identifed as physical and chemical properties, and each substance has these unique properties that allow us to identify it. Physical properties are characteristics that can be determined without a chemical reaction and do not involve chemical changes. Physical properties include color, size, weight, hardness, odor, and gloss. On the other hand, chemical properties are characterized by chemical reactions and chemical changes in the substance. An example of a chemical property or chemical change would be nail enhancements to polymerize or harden.

Again, matter can be changed in two different ways. We think of these different ways as physical forces causing physical changes and chemical reactions causing chemical changes. An example of a physical change occurs when an abrasive file is used on the nail plate and both the nail plate and the file are changed. Another example of a physical change is when nail polish is dissolved and removed with a remover solvent. When you dissolve nail polish in a solvent, it is not a chemical change. Nail polish is made by dissolving certain solid ingredients into a unique blend of solvents which then reform into a solid film as the solvent evaporates away.

A chemical change alters the original chemical composition or makeup of the substance. An example of a chemical change is the polymerization or hardening of nail products to create artificial nail enhancements when exposed to ultraviolet energy. Chemical reactions can release a significant amount of heat and are referred to as exothermic reactions. Nail products that undergo exothermic reactions would be nail enhancements during polymerization. Exothermic reactions occur whenever nail enhancement products polymerize. Normally, the ladies who apply these nail enhancements can't feel the tiny amount of heat being released.

We can classify matter as either a pure

substance or a physical mixture. Pure substances are chemical combinations of a single type of matter. All atoms, elements, molecules and compounds are pure substances. Water is a chemical substance that results from the combination of two hydrogen atoms and one oxygen atom in definite proportions. In fact, liquid water has different physical and chemical properties than hydrogen or oxygen gas. Yet water does not always exist in its natural state. Some water or aqueous solutions could contain chlorine or dissolved minerals. Pure air contains many substances such as nitrogen, oxygen, carbon dioxide, argon, and other gases present in smaller amounts.

A physical mixture is a combination of matter. The properties of the mixture has to do with the properties of each substance in the mixture. Saltwater is a physical mixture of salt and water that dissolves salt in water, and these properties are derived from both the physical and chemical properties of salt and water. Most of the products ladies use are physical mixtures.

We can even further categorize physical mixtures as solutions, suspensions, and emulsions. The differences among them has to do with the size of the particles and the solubility of the substances. A solution can be thought of as a uniform blend of two or more substances. The solute is the substance that dissolves in solution. The solvent is the substance that dissolves the solute and makes up the solution.

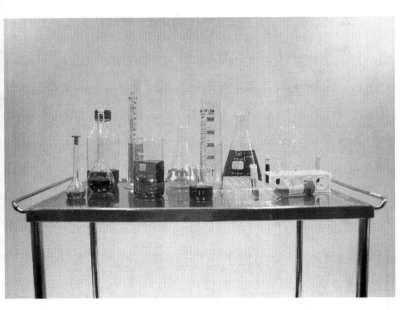

Water is known as the universal solvent because it has the ability to dissolve more substances than any other known substance. Mixing two liquids can be classified as either miscible or immiscible.

Miscible liquids are soluble which means they can be mixed together to form stable solutions. An example would be water and rubbing alcohol or acetone, which is nail polish remover, and water are miscible liquids. Immiscible liquids do not have the ability to be mixed into stable solutions. An example would be water and oil are immiscible liquids. Eventually the two liquids separate from each other and can be visibly observed.

Solutions are soluble mixtures when solid particles are dissolved and the liquid components are soluble. Solutions can be transparent or they can be colored and do not separate from each other when left to stand by itself. As mentioned, salt water is a solution of a solid dissolved in a liquid. Water is considered to be the solvent that dissolves the salt which is the solute and is held in solution. The salt is not a solid anymore because it is now separated and free to move around in water. Artificial nail monomers are solutions that contain dissolved solids and blends of different soluble liquids.

Suspensions are thought of as unstable mixtures of undissolved particles floating around in a liquid. Suspensions contain larger particles that are less miscible than the solution. You can see the particles but they are not large enough to settle quickly to the bottom of the container. Suspensions are not stable and separate over a period of time, and this explains why lotions, creams, and even glitter in nail polish separate in a bottle. Some lotions are suspensions and should be mixed well prior to use. Calamine lotion. liquid mineral makeup, and nail polish are considered to be suspensions.

An emulsion is an unstable physical mixture of two or more substances that do not stay blended without an emulsifier. Emulsifiers bring two different materials together and binds them together, but over time they can separate from each other. It is best to use these cosmetic products within one year to ensure peak performance.

Surfactants which is a contraction for surface active agent are often used as emulsifiers since they act as a bridge to allow oils and water to mix or emulsify and form emulsions. Surfactants have two distinct parts which includes the head of the surfactant molecule known as being hydrophilic. Hydrophilic means water loving. The tail of the surfactant is known as being lipophilic which means oil loving. The hydrophilic head dissolves in water whereas the lipophilic tail dissolves in oil. Furthermore, surfactant molecules mix and dissolve in both oil and water and links them together to form an emulsion.

There are two types of emulsions that I like to discuss. The first one is oil-in-water (O/W) emulsion where oil droplets are emulsified in water. The droplets of oil are surrounded by surfactants where the lipophilic tails point inward toward the center of the droplet. The tiny droplets form an O/W emulsion because the oil is surrounded by water. Note that oil-in-water emulsions do not feel as greasy as water-in-oil (W/O) emulsions. The oil has a lower concentration than the water and hides by the surfactant molecules in which it surrounds. Most of the emulsions that are used in salons are oil-in-water, and examples of these would be lotions and creams.

In a water-in-oil emulsion, there are water droplets being emulsified in oil. The droplets of water are surrounded by surfactants with the hydrophilic heads pointing inward. There are tiny droplets of water that form the internal portion of the W/O emulsion because water is completely surrounded by oil. Water-in-oil emulsions feel more greasier than oil-in-water emulsions since the water is hidden and the oil forms the external portion of the emulsion. Foot balms are considered to be water-in-oil emulsions.

There are other types of physical mixtures. Ointments, pomades, pastes, and styling waxes are considered to be semisolid mixtures made with combinations of petrolatum, oil, and wax. Powders are also considered to be physical mixtures of one or more different types of solids. White or colored polymer powders are mixtures of powders and pigments.

There are common ingredients in products. Volatile alcohols are alcohols that evaporate easily and include isopropyl alcohol or rubbing alcohol and ethyl alcohol. On the other hand, fatty alcohols such as cetyl alcohol and cetearyl alcohol are nonvolatile alcohol waxes that are used as skin conditioners. Glycerin is a sweet, colorless, and oily substance that is used as a solvent and as a moisturizer in skin and body creams. Silicones are used in nail polish dryers and as skin protectants, and there are volatile organic compounds or volatile organic solvents such as ethyl acetate and isopropyl alcohol that is used in nail polish, base and top coats, and even nail polish removers.

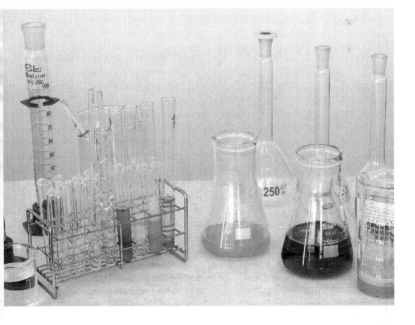

Let us wrap this first chapter and talk about potential hydrogen. Potential hydrogen or pH is discussed with reference to salon products. The small "p" represents a quantity and the capital H represents the hydrogen ion. An ion is an atom or a molecule that carries an electrical charge, and ionization causes an atom or molecule to split in two to create a pair of ions with opposite electrical charges.

An ion with a negative electrical charge is considered to be an anion. An ion with a positive electrical charge is considered to be a cation. In water, some of the water molecules ionize into hydrogen ions, H^+, and hydroxide ions, OH^-, where we can use the pH scale to measure these ions. The hydrogen ion is considered to be acidic. If there are more hydrogen ions in solution, then the more acidic the solution would be. The hydroxide anion is known to be alkaline or basic. The more hydroxide anions present in solution, the more basic the solution will be. We can measure pH because of the ionization of water. Products that contain water can have pH of around 7. Pure water is considered to be neutral because it contains an equal number of hydrogen cations and hydroxide anions.

The pH scale measures acidity and alkalinity of a substance and has a range of 0 to 14. If the pH becomes less than 7, then the solution is acidic. On the other hand, if the pH becomes greater than 7, then the solution is basic. The equation for pH is

$$pH = -\log[OH^-]$$

Even though pure water has a pH of 7, it

is not neutral to the hair and skin which has an average pH of 5. In fact, pure water can cause the hair to swell as much as 20% and can be drying to the skin.

Again, acids produce hydrogen cations which we actually refer to as hydronium cations. They have a pH less than 7 and can turn litmus paper from blue to red which is the opposite of a basic solution that can turn litmus paper from red to blue. Alpha hydroxy acids or AHA are acids encountered in salons. Citric acid is used to adjust the pH of a lotion or cream.

Alkalis produce hydroxide anions, and they feel slippery and soapy on the skin Alkalis soften and swell the cuticle on the nail plate and even on callused skin. Sodium hydroxide which is written as the chemical symbols NaOH is also used as a callus softener. One should be cautious using callus softeners since they have high pH values. These products should not be used on living skin since they can cause injury to the hands and feet and may lead to painful skin burn and irritation. If you mix an acid and a base, you always form a salt and water which is called a neutralization reaction. We can represent this reaction as follows:

$$Acid + Base \rightarrow Salt + Water$$

In other words when we mix hydrogen cations and hydroxide anions, they neutralize each other to form water. In fact, liquid soaps are slightly acidic and can help alkaline callus softener and remove any residues that is left on the skin after rinsing with water.

I like to wrap up this chapter and talk about color theory since ladies love the blend of different colors in nail polishes. Visible light is also called electromagnetic radiation that we see. Electromagnetic radiation is also called radiant energy because it radiates energy through space by waves. The distance between two successive peaks or troughs is called wavelength. Wavelength and frequency have an inverse relationship. Long wavelengths have low frequency which means the number of waves is fewer within a given length. Short wavelengths have higher frequency because there are more waves within a given length.

When we look at the visible spectrum of light, violet has the shortest wavelength and red has the longest wavelength. The wavelength of ulraviolet radiation is above violet, and it is above the visible spectrum of light. But remember that infrared and ultraviolet rays are not light at all. They are wavelengths of electromagnetic radiation beyond the visible spectrum. Ultraviolet-cured nail enhancements make use of ultraviolet radiation which is electromagnetic radiation with a wavelength shorter than visible light and longer than X-rays. We cannot see these frequencies, but they are visible to insects and birds. Ultraviolet radiation have shorter wavelengths, but more energy, and it does not penetrate as deep as visible light.

We can summarize the relationships of energy, wavelength, and frequency as follows: $E = hv$ or $E = hc / \lambda$ where $v = c / \lambda$. The designation E stands for energy, h is Planck's contant and has the value of

6.626 x 10^{-34} J*s, v pronounced nu and is frequency, λ is lambda and is wavelength, and c is the speed of light and has the value of 3.00 x 10^8 m/s. You can see that energy is directly proportional to frequency and inversely proportional to wavelength.

Remember you need to protect ultraviolet curing products from light. Nail enhancement products are exposed to sunlight or artificial room lighting can cure the container which in turn becomes less effective. Heating can cause the solution to discolor while it is still in the original container.

Based on our understanding of wavelengths, freqency, and energy, we can explain why we see different colors in our everday life. White light or sunlight contains all of the colors of light (red, orange, yellow, green, blue, violet). When we see red nail polish, for example, it actually absorbs all of the colors except the color which it appears as red. This is why we see red. Remember all colors have specific wavelengths from 400 nanometers which is blue-violet to 700 nanometers which is red. It is the wavelength of the color we see based on the absorption of the rest of the colors by the object.

<u>Color</u> <u>Wavelength</u>

Red 630 - 750 nm

Orange 590 - 630 nm

Yellow 570 - 590 nm

Green 490 - 570 nm

Blue 450 - 490 nm

Indigo 420 - 450 nm

Violet 380 - 420 nm

Color wheels illustrate and identify primary, secondary, tertiary, and complementary colors. Again, the light we observe from a surface is called color. As mentioned already, red nail polish appears red since red light is reflecting off its surface. We see black when there is no color reflecting from its surface. This is why black nail polish absorbs light that hits its surface and none of it is reflected back to our eyes. In fact, nail polish looks white when all colors are reflected. The colors we see depends on which colors are reflected and which colors are absorbed.

Primary colors are considered to be pure pigment colors that can't be obtained from mixing other colors together. They are pure colors and can be modified into different shades by mixing either with black or white. Primary colors are red, yellow, and blue. Secondary colors result from mixing equal parts of two primary colors together. They sit opposite the primary colors on the color wheel. Secondary colors include orange which is a combination of red and yellow, green which is a combination of yellow and blue, and violet which is a combination of blue and red. Tertiary colors or intermediate colors result from mixing a primary color and one of its nearest secondary colors. They include red-orange, red-violet, blue-green, yellow-green, and yellow-orange.

Complementary colors are colors located opposite each other on the color wheel. If you mix together equal parts, they produce a neutral brown color. When mixed in unequal parts, they produce a neutral color that is dominated by the color of the greatest amount. Applying these complementary colors side by side enhances each other and makes them stand out. You can see why ladies like to explore these great color combinations and different shades and designs of nail polish.

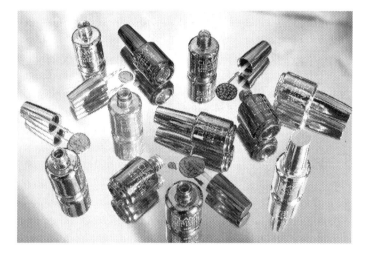

Chapter 2

Nail Tips and Wraps

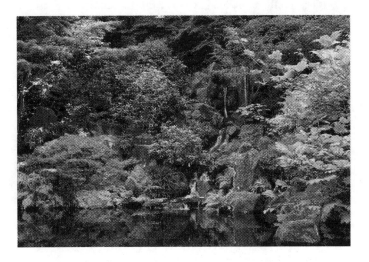

Ladies love to wear beautiful nails in an endless variety of lengths and strengths. It does not matter to some ladies whether they are wearing long, medium, or short nails. She might have nail tips applied over her natural nails based on strength and durability. Once a tip is applied, she has the opportunity to choose from so many products that can be layered over her natural nail and tip to secure the strength of the nail and at the same time to stay beautiful.

Nail tips are considered to be plastic and premolded nails shaped from a tough polymer made of acrylonitrile butadiene styrene (ABS) plastic. They can be adhered to the natural nail so extra length can be added and to serve as a support for nail enhancement products. These tips can be combined with an overlay which is a layer of a kind of nail enhancement product applied over the tip for added strength. Note that nail tips that don't have an overlay are not long wearing and can break easily.

Along with the basic materials of your

manicure table, you are going to need a abrasive board, a buffer block, a tip adhesive, a tip cutter, an implement similar to a nail clipper that is designed for use on nail tips, a nail dehydrator which is a substance used to remove surface moisture and small amounts of oil left on the natural nail plate, and of course a variety of nail tips for nail tip application.

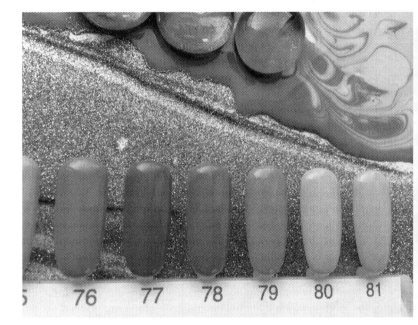

Many nail tips have shallow depressions called a well that serves as a contact point with the nail plate. There is a position stop which is the point where the free edge of the natural nail meets the tip, and it is the point where the tip is adhered to the nail. There are many kinds of nail tips that includes the partial well, the full well, and the well-less.

When taking the time to apply a tip that has a well, you need to be sure that the well butts up against the natural nail when it adheres to the nail. Nail tips come in many different sizes, colors, and shapes so that it is easier to fit on your nails. When choosing tips, the nail plate needs to be covered from sidewall to sidewall exactly. Do not use a nail tip that is narrower than the nail plate. As the nail plate grows, the natural nail will be considered to be wider and get caught in hair or clothes etc. In fact, the tip may also crack at the sides and split down the middle. So don't use a too-small tip on the nail. It is better to use a slightly larger tip and work with an abrasive board to work with the tip before applying it. It is also possible to trim and bevel the well area before applying the tip to the nail which saves blending time. Keep in mind that nail tips are prebeveled which require less filing on the natural nail after application. This helps lesson the potential for damage to the natural nail.

The bonding agent that is used to secure the nail tip to the natural nail is called a nail tip adhesive. "Gel adhesives" are sometimes referred to as resin and are the thickest and require more time to dry than fast-setting thinner adhesives and only dry in about five seconds. Be very careful when using adhesives because even the smallest amount of adhesive in the eyes is dangerous and causes serious injury. Once the nail tips are applied, the contact area needs to be reduced with an abrasive so the tip blends with the natural nail. With perfect tip applications, there should be no visible line where the natural nail stops and the tip starts to begin.

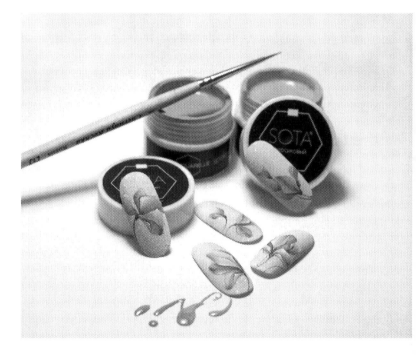

Any procedure that secures a layer of fabric and around the nail tip to ensure strength and durability is called a nail wrap. Nail wraps can be thought of as overlays that can be used over nail tips, and they are used to repair and strengthen natural nails to create nail extensions. Nail wraps describe any overlay that includes a nail wrap resin to coat and secure fabric wraps to the natural nail and nail tip. Wrap resins are actually made from cyanoacrylate which is an adhesive and which is closely related to other kinds of nail enhancements.

A fabric wrap made of silk, linen, or fiberglass are popular nail wraps because of its durability. Fabric wraps are cut to cover the surface of the natural nail and the nail tip. It is also laid onto a layer of wrap resin to strengthen the enhancement. Once again, nail wraps are used as an overlay to strengthen natural nails and to strengthen the nail tip application.

A silk wrap is made from thin natural material with a tight weave that becomes transparent when wrap resin gets applied. Note that a silk wrap is lightweight and contains a smooth appearance when applied to the nail. A linen wrap is made from closely woven and heavy material. It is thicker and bulkier than other types of wrap fabrics. Note that wrap adhesives don't penetrate linen as much as silk or fiberglass. Linen wraps are opaque so a colored polish should be used to cover it completely even after wrap resin gets applied. Linen is preferred to be used since it is considered to be a strong wrap fabric. A fiberglass wrap is made from a thin synthetic mesh with a loose weave. This loose weave makes it easy to use and allows the wrap resin to penetrate and improves adhesion and clarity. Note that fiberglass is not as strong as silk or linen, but it does create durable nail enhancements. Paper wraps are no longer used since it lacks strength and durability.

A wrap resin accelerator or an activator is used as the dryer that speeds up the hardening process of the wrap resin or adhesive overlay. Activators come in different forms such as a brush-on bottle, pump spray-on, and aerosol. Activators dissipate in about two minutes after being applied so do not reapply additional wrap resin immediately or you might find the activator to cause the resin to harden on the brush, tip of the bottle, or extended when it touches the nail. Note that activators do not need to be applied after every layer of adhesive. Activators can be used as need

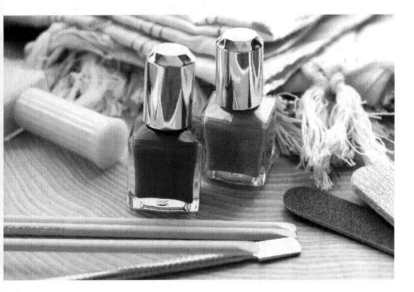

When choosing wrap material, you are going to need a wrap resin, resin accelerator, nail buffer and file, small scissors, plastic, and tweezers to carry out a nail wrap overlay. If you use a flexible plastic sheet to press fabric onto the nail plate, it prevents the transfer of oil and debris from your fingers. Wrap resins don't easily penetrate fibers that are contaminated with oil. The strands become visible in the clear coating. It is a good idea to not touch them more than you can. You will need to change an unused portion of the plastic for each of your fingers when necessary.

Now it comes to the point about maintaining, repairing, and removing nail wraps. Fabric wraps need to be maintained regularly so they can be kept looking fresh. Nail wraps should have consistent maintenance after being applied. Maintenance is carried out when a nail enhancement needs to be serviced after two or more weeks from the initial application of the nail enhancement product. Maintaining the nail wrap accomplishes the goal to apply the enhancement product onto the new growth of the nail which is commonly called a fill or a backfill and to correct the nail to ensure its strength, shape, and durability which is referred to as rebalance. Wrap maintenance is carried out with either additional wrap resin for the two-week fabric wrap maintenance or with fabric and resin as in the four-week fabric wrap maintenance.

Keep in mind that fabric wrap repair may need to be carried out at times. Small pieces of fabric is used to strengthen a weak point in the nail or to repair a break found in the nail. A stress strip is a strip of fabric cut to a about 3.12 mm in length and applied to a weak point of the nail. This takes place during the four-week maintenance to repair or strengthen a specific weak point in a nail enhancement. A repair patch, on the other hand, is a piece of fabric cut to completely cover either a crack or a break in the nail. Again you would want to use the four week fabric wrap maintenance procedure to apply a repair patch.

There is going to be a time when you want your nail wraps removed. The wraps need to be carefully removed to make sure the nail plate is not damaged. Nail wraps are removed by immersing the wrap enhancement into a small bowl filled with acetone. Acetone has the chemical formula C_3H_6O with a carbonyl and two methyl groups chemically bonded to both ends of the carbonyl. The polar and nonpolar character of acetone has its ability to remove the nail wrap. The nail wrap gets melted away and then carefully and gently slide the softened wrap material away from the nail with a wooden pusher. I would suggest to have a manicure after the enhancement is removed to rehydrate the natural nail and cuticle.

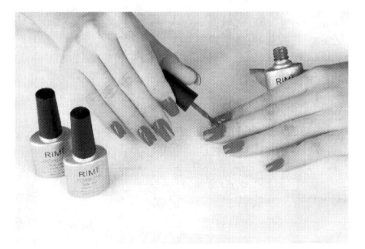

Chapter 3

Nail Enhancements

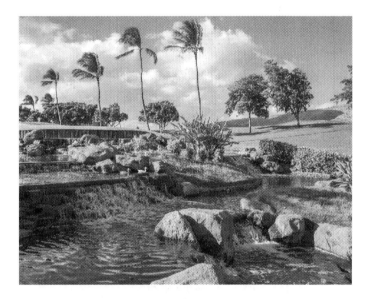

Nail enhancements are based on mixing together liquids and powders and are referred to as acrylic. Acrylic refers to an entire family of thousands of different substances that share closely related features. In fact, acrylics are used to make contact lenses, Plexiglas Windows, cements for fixing broken bones, makeup, and other cosmetics. Just about all nail enhancement products are based on ingredients that come from the acrylic family.

Ingredients found in two-part monomer liquid and polymer powder enhancement systems belong to the acrylic family called "methacrylates". We can think of acrylic as a general term for a large group of ingredients. Interestingly, monomer liquids and polymer powders come in many different colors such as variations of pink, white, clear, and natural. The colors can be used by themselves or blended to create different shades the color of your desire usually pink for the nail bed and which can be used for a wide range of designs and patterns. By using these powders, a unique set of colors and designs can be part of the nail enhancement. You can even use monomer liquid and polymer powder nail enhancements with a single color powder if you decide to wear nail polish all the time or you can create it by using a pink or natural-colored powder over the nail bed and a soft white powder to show a natural nail free edge. You can even use a white powder to give that French manicure look, and even then finish the nail enhancement by polishing the nail to give a high-glossy shine.

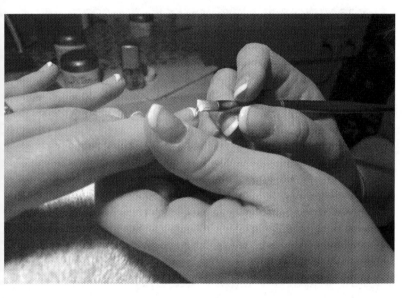

Monomer liquid and polymer powder nail enhancements are also known as sculptured nails. They are created by mixing monomer liquid with a polymer powder. The powder can be white, clear, pink, and many other colors to make the nail enhancement. The word monomer can be broken down to mean mono which means one and mer which means units. We can think of monomer as one unit or one molecule. The prefix poly means many, so when we use the word polymer, it means many units or many molecules linked together in a chain. Both monomer liquid and polymer powder products can either be applied as on the natural nail and as a protective overlay over a nail tip, on a specific form to create a nail extension, or even on small works of art that can be on top or inside a nail enhancement.

You can use a natural brush to apply these nail enhancement products. You would put the brush in a monomer liquid where the natural hair bristle absorb the monomer liquid. Then the tip of the brush is touched to the surface of the dry polymer powder. As the monomer liquid absorbs the polymer powder, a small bead of a product tends to form. The small bead is placed on the nail surface and is then molded into the shape of the brush. The monomer liquid portion could either be ethyl methacrylate, methyl methacrylate, or odorless monomer liquid. Normally, ethyl methacrylate and odorless monomer liquid is used. Methyl methacrylate is illegal in some states because nail products don't adhere well to the nail plate causing the nail to shred and thin the nail plate, creates rigid nail enhancements and if it gets jammed, the overly filed and thinned natural plate breaks before the nail enhancement that can also lead to serious damage, is difficult to remove, and final the Federal Drug Administration (FDA) states don't use it.

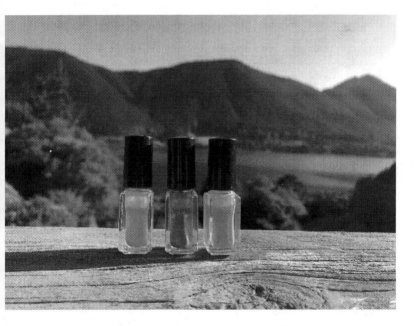

Again, the polymer powder is made mainly from ethyl methacrylate monomer liquid. The polymer powder is made by polymerization which is also known as curing or hardening. it is a chemical reaction that creates polymers. Over trillions of monomers are linked together to create long chains. The long chains create tiny round beads of polymer powder with different sizes. They are poured through a series of special screens where the beads by size are sorted. The right size are then separated and mixed with other special additives and colorants. The final mixture is then packaged and sold as polymer powder.

Special additives are mixed into both the liquid and powder to make sure there is a complete set, maximum durability, color stability, and shelf life. The custom additives is what makes the product work. The polymer powders are mixed with pigments and colorants to make a lot of different shades including pink, whites, and milky translucent shades. There can be even different shades of reds, blues, greens, purples, yellows, oranges, browns, and black.

When liquid gets picked up by a brush and is then mixed with the powder, the bead forms on the end of the brush which quickly begins to harden. It is then placed with other beads and shaped into place while they harden. For the process to begin, the monomers and polymers need additives called catalysts. Catalysts can be elements, compounds, or molecules designed to speed up a reaction without itself being consumed. They are added to the monomer liquid and used to control the curing time. When the monomer liquid and polymer powder are combined with each other, the catalyst that is in the liquid controls the hardening time. Catalysts energizes and activates initiators.

Initiators that are in the polymer powder and when they get activated by a catalyst will cause the monomer molecules to link together into long polymer chains. This is what we call the polymerization process. Polymerization starts when the liquid in the brush picks up powder from the container and forms a bead. Forming polymers is like a chain reaction or what we call a polymerization reaction. It is a process that joins together monomers to make long polymer chains.

The initiator, that is added to the polymer powder, is the molecule called benzoyl peroxide which is abbreviated as BPO. BPO is used to start the chain reaction which leads to curing or hardening of the nail enhancement. Different types of nail enhancements have different concentrations of BPO where some of the monomer liquids require more BPO to cure than others. It is critical to use polymer powder designed for the monomer liquid that you plan to use. You don't want to use the wrong powder to make the nail enhancement or that might lead to skin irritation or sensivity.

Monomer liquids need to be combined with polymer powders to form nail enhancements. The amount of monomer liquid and polymer powder can be used to make a bead and is called the mix ratio. The bead mix ratio is described as dry, medium, or wet. If there are equal amounts of liquid and powder used to create the bead, we call it a dry bead. If there is twice as much liquid as powder to create the bead, we call it a wet bead. One-and-a-half more liquid than powder is called a medium bead. In general, medium beads are the best and ideal mixing ratio when working with monomer liquids and polymer powders.

The mix ratio makes sure there is a proper set and maximum durability for the nail enhancement. If there is too much powder that is picked up in the bead, the nail enhancement will lead to brittleness and discoloration. If there is too little powder picked up in the bead, the nail enhancement becomes weak and there will be a risk of developing skin irritation and sensitivity around the skin might increase. But the nice thing about polymer powder is that it is available in a wide variety of colors such as white, clear, natural, pink, and many other colors. You decide which nail enhancement you like to use at a salon.

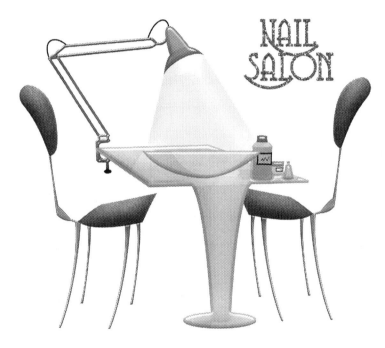

Let us now talk about nail dehydrators. Nail dehydrators have the ability to remove surface moisture and tiny amounts of oil that is left on the natural nail plate and which has the ability to block adhesion. You should use the nail dehydrator liberally to the natural plate only. Skin contact needs to be avoided. After the dehydrator is dried, it is best not to touch the nail plate before applying any primer.

Nail primers are used on the natural nail before applying product to assist in adhesion. The primer is used to chemically bond the nail enhancement product to the natural nail. One of the ends of the primer molecule chemically bonds to the nail protein in the natural nail. On the other end of the molecule is a methacrylate that bonds to the monomer liquid as it cures.

There are two kinds of nail primers for a monomer liquid and polymer powder nail enhancement. These include acid-based and nonacid or acid-free primers. Acid-based nail primers such as methacrylic acid can be used to help adhere enhancements to the natural nail. However, the nail primer is corrosive to the skin and dangerous to the eyes so acid-free and nonacid primers are used instead. Still make sure skin contact should be avoided during application.

The applicator brush should be inserted into the nail primer. Any excess should be wiped from the brush. Use a slightly damp brush and completely cover the nail plate with the primer. It is not a good idea to use too much product or it can run onto the skin and cause skin irritation and sensitivity. The brush needs to hold enough product to prepare two or three nails. Finally before dipping the brush back inside the container, make sure you wipe the brush on a clean disposable table towel. This way you don't contaminate the bottle with any debris the brush could have picked up. Do not apply nail enhancement product over wet nail primer. This causes product discoloration and service breakdown. Make sure you only apply primer to the natural nail. Do not put nail primer on plastic nail tips.

Let us continue our discussion and now talk about abrasives. Abrasives are used to describe nail files and buffers. They have a grit number which refers to how many grains of sand are on the file per square inch. The lower the number means the rougher the abrasive will be. The higher the number, the softer it will be. Different abrasive core materials change how an abrasive will work. Plastic and wood cores can be used for files and plastics, whereas sponge cores can be used in buffers. Wood makes the abrasive more aggressive, whereas the sponge core forms around the nail core and is gentle.

Common abrasives that are used for filing, shaping, and buffing nail enhancements include a course-grit file, a medium-grit file, a fine-grit file or buffer, or a shiner. A course-grit file is 100 grit or lower and is strong enough to thin enhancement product to prepare the enhancement for rebalance. Make sure you avoid using coarser and lower-grit abrasives on nail enhancement products as they can damage the created nail enhancement.

A medium-grit file is 150 to 180 grit and is used for initial shaping of the perimeter of the nail. It is also used for refining the overall surface shape for the nail enhancement and for smoothing the surface before buffing. If you do your best to avoid putting the product on too thick, you can use a 180 grit which is strong enough to shape the entire nail enhancement. You can also use a fine-grit file or buffer which is 240 grit or higher. It is used to finish filing, refining, and buffing. The grit of the file is used to shape the free edge of a natural nail. A shiner is a buffer which is usually 400/1000/4000 and is used to create a high shine on a natural nail or a nail enhancement when there is no polish being worn. The buffer has three sides. You have to buff the entire nail with the lowest grit side first and then repeat the other sides to create that glossy shine to the nail itself. In fact, shiner buffers can also only have two sides. You could buff the entire surface of the nail with a 240- or 350-grit buffer before buffing with the shiner.

Nail forms are placed under the free edge of your natural nails. It is used as a guide to extend nail enhancements that are beyond the fingertips for more length. There are disposbale nail forms that are made of paper or Mylar which is coated with adhesive backs. There are also reusable nail forms that are made of preshaped plastic or aluminum which can also be cleaned and disinfected.

Nail tips are preformed nail extensions that are made from acrylonitrile butadiene styrene (ABS) or tenite acetate plastic. They come in a wide variety of shapes, styles, and color such as natural, white, and clear. Nail tips can be adhered to the tip of the natural nail with a fast set resin so the length can be extended. However, they are not strong enough to wear by themselves so they have to be overlaid with enhancement products.

Both the monomer liquid and polymer powder are each poured into a special dish which we call a dappen dish. These types of dishes have narrow openings to minimize the evaporation of the monomer liquid into the air. It is not a good idea to use open mouth jars or containers with large openings. They increase evaporation of the liquid and allow the product to be contaminated with air particles. It is important that a dappen dish should be covered with a tightly fit lid when it is not in use.

Each time the brush gets dipped into the dappen dish, the remaining monomer liquid gets contaminated with small amounts of polymer powder. It is never a good idea to pour any unused portion of monomer liquid back to the original container. Make sure you empty the monomer liquid from the dappen dish after using it and then wipe it clean with a disposable towel. To make sure there is no skin irritation or sensitivity, don't contact the skin with the monomer liquid during this process, and make sure you wipe the dish clean with acetone before storing it in a place where there is no dust.

The nail brush is just as important in this whole process in creating a nail enhancement. Best nail brushes to use with monomer liquid and polymer powder enhancement products are composed of natural kolinsky, sable, or a blend of both. The brushes can be oval, round, or square and come in many different sizes. A most common used brush for monomer liquid and polymer powder is a #8 oval brush. Avoid using synthetic and less expensive brushes since they do not pick up enough monomer liquid and do not release the liquid in a proper fashion. It is also a good idea to avoid overly large brushes usually the size of 12 to 16 since they hold excessive amounts of liquid and alter the mix ratio of the powder and liquid. Plus the disadvantage using the large size is that it allows the brush to touch the skin during the application which then overexposes yourself to the monomer which leads to the risk of developing skin irritations or sensitivities. Odorless monomer liquids require less liquid so using a flat brush holds less liquid and is best recommended.

When you are done using these products, store monomer liquid and polymer powder products in a covered container. You should also store all primers and liquids separate from each other and preferably in a cool and dark area so light does not react with these monomers. Avoid storing them near heat since heat can decompose the monomers into new products. Make sure you never save monomer liquid removed from the original container. Pour it into a very absorbent paper towel and put it in a plastic bag. Make sure to avoid skin contact with the monomer liquid and don't pour it directly into the plastic bag, or it will react with the plastic bag. If the monomer liquid gets on your skin, please make sure you wash your hands with liquid soap and water. Make sure you collect all used materials and seal them in a plastic bag to be put into a closed waste receptacle.

Now comes the point where you want to maintain the nail enhancement to the best you possiblly can. Taking time for regular maintenance helps prevent nail enhancements from lifting or cracking. If you don't take the time to maintain your nail enhancement, then there is a greater tendency for lifting, cracking, or bending and breaking. This can lead to you developing an infection or having other health problems. A qualified nail technician at a salon will repair the nail enhancement by filling the area and adding monomer liquid and polymer powder to it which is called crack repair.

Normally clients who visit the salon will carry out this proper maintenance every two to three weeks which also depends how fast the client's nails grow. The nail enhancement is basically thinned down to blend with new growth area for the natural nail. The apex of the nail is then filed away, and the entire nail enhancement gets reduced in thickness which is then prepared for an overlay of new product.

Let us get a little deeper into this topic on properly structured nail enhancements. Remember your nail enhancements need to look good and remain strong and healthy. The apex is also known as the arch, and it is the area of the nail that has the most strength. Strength in the apex allows the base of the nail, sidewalls, and tip to be thin and leaves the nail strong enough to resist breaking. The apex is oval shapped, and it is located in the center of the nail.

The stress area is the place where the natural nail grows beyond the finger tip and also becomes the free edge. The area needs strength to support the extension. The sidewall is the area on the side of the nail plate which grows free of its natural attachment to the nail fold, and it is also where the extension leaves the nail. The nail extension underside is the underside of the nail extension. This nail extension underside is straight out or may dip depending on the nail style. The undersides need to be even and match the length from nail to nail in all of the fingers. The tip itself should fit the nail and finger properly. Even the underside of the nail extension is supposed to be smooth without any glitches. It is also important that the thickness of the nail enhancement should be thin if you are going to wear it comfortably. The nail enhancement itself should graduate from the cuticle area to the end of the nail extension so you don't feel an edge. I think of the sidewalls and tip's edge to be as thin as a credit card. There is also a C curve of the nail enhancement which also depends on the C curve of the natural nail. The top surface portion and bottom surface portion needs to be matched perfectly. Salons and spas recommend a 35% C-curve to be the average. The C-curve provides structure to the nail so it can look slender on the hand. Remember that C-curves provide strength. Finally, you need to make sure the lengths of the nail extensions and enhancements are even. You need to measure the length of the index, middle, and ring fingers, and these should be the same length. Of course, do not forget the pinkie and thumb fingers need to also be in proportion and match.

At this point, you might be wondering

about the nail enhancement removal process so let us talk about it. Soak the nail enhancements off of the nails using acetone or a solution recommended by the manufacturer. Odorless monomer liquid and polymer powder products don't have the same chemistry as other monomer liquid and polymer powder products. The products do not rely on ethyl acrylic and rely on monomers that have little odor. Although they are called odorless, they have a slight odor or low odor.

In general, odorless products must be used with dry mixing ratios or equal parts of liquid and powder in a bead. If they are too wet when being applied, you risk developing skin irritation or sensitivity. The mix ratio creates a bead that looks like frost on the brush. After it is placed on the nail, it slowly forms into a firm glossy bead that holds its shape until pressed and smooth with the nail brush. You need to make sure you brush frequently so the product does not stick to the hairs. It is not a good idea to rewet the brush with monomer liquid. This changes the mix ratio and leads to product discoloration and increased risk of skin irritation and sensitivity. Without re-wetting the brush, make sure you use it to shape and smooth the surface to being perfect.

Odorless products tend to harden more slowly and creates a tacky layer which we call an inhabitation layer. The layer can be rolled off or filed away with a 150-grit abrasive used fom cuticle to free edge. Make sure you avoid skin contact with these particles. In fact, some of the manufacturers make a resin that brushes on to cure the tacky layer and must be applied immediately after creating the nail enhancement. This creates a hard surface on the odorless product which makes it filing and shaping more easier. Above all, let us not forget colored polymer powder products. There are polymer powders that are available in a variety of colors with almost every shade of nail polish which adds greater chemistry and greater beauty to nails.

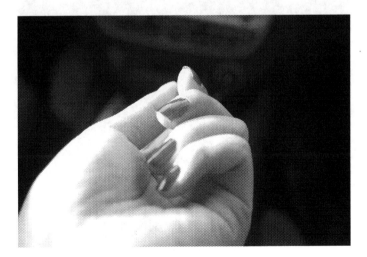

Chapter 4

Different Gels

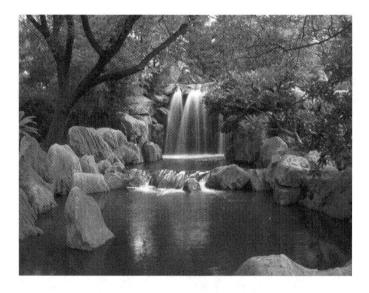

Ultraviolet gels is a type of nail enhancement product that has the ability to harden when exposed to a UV light source. UV gel enhancements contain ingredients from the monomer and polymer chemical family.

The ingredients are part of a subcategory of family called acrylates and methacrylates. There are wrap resins that are called cyanoacrylates, and there are monomer liquid/polymer nail enhancements from the same category as UV gels that are called methacrylates.

Harminder Gill

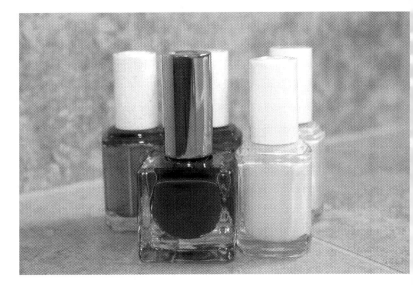

UV and LED gels contain monomers, but they rely on a related form called an oligomer. Oligomers are short chain monomers that are long enough to be referred to as a prepolymer. They are often thick, gel-like, and sticky. Urethane acrylate and urethane methacrylate are main ingredients that are used to create UV gel nail enhancements. Urethanes are known for high abrasion resistance and durability.

UV gel resins react with UV light where a photoinitiator causes the polymerization reaction to begin. The resin, photoinitiator, and the proper curing lamp causes the gel to cure. The single component resin compound is cured to a solid material when exposed to a UV light source. Remember it takes the resin, photoinitiator, and the proper curing lamp to make the get cure. UV gel systems have a single component resin compound that gets cured to a solid material when it is exposed to a UV light source. Both UV and LED gels do not use a powder that is found in the gel resin. A few UV gels incorporate a powder that is sprinkled into the gel. Both UV and LED gels can be applied, filed, and maintained. What is nice about them is they have little to no odor. They are not, however, as hard as monomer and polymer nail enhancements, but they can look nice and are long-lasting nail enhancements. The application process of UV and LED gel enhancements are different than other nail enhancements. After preparing the nail plate, each layer of product that is applied to the natural nail and nail tip will require an exposure to UV or LED light to harden. The light from the lamp emits a proper type and intensity of light.

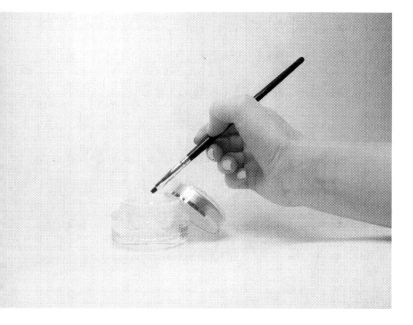

Some of the ladies prefer UV gels that are thick, whereas other ladies prefer UV gels that self-level quickly. Either way we can describe different UV gels being thin-viscosity gels, medium-viscosity gels, thick-viscosity gels, and building or sculpting gels. Viscosity can be thought of as a measurement of the thickness or thinness of a liquid where it affects how a fluid flows. Some manufacturers have a market name for UV gels. Most UV gels fall under the general categories as a one-color method or a two-color method. Clear resins are used for the one-color method for clients who wish to wear colored polish or gel polish over the enhancement. Pink-resin and white-pigmented resin are used for the two-color method who prefer the French or American manicure finish without any nail lacquer. Each manufacturer have their own specific instructions how to carry out each process. Make sure you keep the brush and gel away from sunlight, UV, LED gel lamps, and full-spectrum table lamps that prevent gels from hardening. After using the equipment, store the application brush away from sources of UV light. Do not have a container of gel open near light otherwise the gel will cure and polymerize in the container.

UV bonding gels increase adhesion to the natural nail plate, but they vary in consistency and chemical components. Adhesion decreases nail enhancements to separate from the natural nail plate. UV building gels contain thick viscosity resin that allows a nail professional to build an arch and curve to the fingernail. These kind of gels are used with self-leveling UV gels that reduce the amount of filing and shaping to contour the enhancement. There are UV building gels that have fiberglass strands that are part of the gel. These UV gels have hardness and durability properties. They are also helpful when nail technicians repair a break or crack in a client's enhancement.

UV self-leveling gels enhance the thickness of other gels which provides a smoother surface than some UV building gels. Normally nail techncians will apply a UV building gel during their service first and then a self-leveling gel during the second part of the service that reduces filing and contouring at a later time. Pigmented gels are building gels or self-leveling gels that also contains pigments. Building style of pigmented gels are used earlier during the service since they are used to create a two color process. Self-leveling pigmented UV and LED gels are used near the final contouring procedure whether it is before or after the contouring. They are applied more thinly than pigmented building gels and require little of any filing. Pigmented gels vary in opacity and viscosity. Normally, more opaque gels have thinner viscosities that are applied after the second coat of a building gel. Less opaque pigmented gels are thicker in viscosity and are applied before the first coat of a building gel. Gel polishes are alternative to traditional nail laquers, and they get cured in the lamp. Once the gel polish is finished curing, a gloss gel can be applied over it to create a high lustrous shine. Even gel polishes can be used on natural nails. Gel polishes come in a lot of colors and even in cream and frosted colors, and some of them include glitter.

UV gloss gels are also called sealing gels, finished gels, or shine gels. These gels do not require buffing and can be used over monomer and polymer enhancement. There are two types of UV and LED gloss gels. Traditional gloss gels cure with a sticky inhibition layer which requires cleaning. Tack-free gloss gels cure to a high shine without the inhibition layer. Inhibition layers consist of a tacky surface left on the nail after the UV gel has cured. It is best to choose a gloss gel of your liking. Traditional UV gloss gels do not discolor after prolonged exposure to UV light. Learning how each gel behaves on the fingernail is good since now you can learn how to use pink gels and whole gels. Both pink gels and white gels can be formulated in a variety of viscosities and opacities.

Requirements for UV and LED gel supplies include UV or LED gel lamp, small, flat, or oval nylon bristles, UV or LED gel primer or bonding gel, UV or LED gel, nail tips with the right curves to your fingernail, nail adhesive, nail cleaner, abrasive files and buffers such as a medium abrasive 180 grit for natural nail preparation, a fine abrasive 240 grit that is used for smoothing, and a fine buffer 350 grit or higher for finishing, and lint-free cleansing wipes.

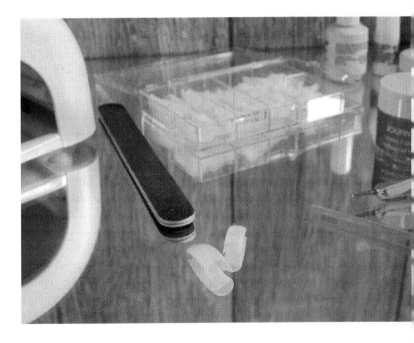

Know that gels have fewer odors than acrylics. The choice of whether to use a gel polish versus a traditional polish depends on you. If you prefer to have the polish removed outside of the salon, then a traditional polish might be better. If you prefer the polish to remain on the fingernail for two weeks, then consider a gel polish.

Choosing the proper UV or LED gel is important. If you have flat fingernails, then more building will be needed to create an arch and a curve. Building is easier when using thicker UV building gel. If you have fingernails that have an arch and curve, then a self-leveling gel will work best. You want to choose a self-leveling gel that works best for you whether it is medium- or thick-viscosity gel. If you get broken enhancements, then you may want to get a gel that uses fiberglass at your next salon visit.

A UV or LED bulb emits light to cure gel nail enhancements. These bulbs vary in curing power. A UV or LED lamp is also considered to be a light unit and which controls UV and LED bulbs to cure gel nail enhancements. They affect the curing power of the unit. Lamps are referred to by the bulbs inside the lamp multiplied by wattage. A unit of wattage is a measure of how much electricity the lamp consumes. Wattage does not tell us how much UV light a UV lamp will emit. Different lamps produce varying amounts of UV light. This is referred to as UV light intensity or concentration. You want to use a UV lamp designed for the selected UV gel product. UV bulbs can stay violet for years, but after a few months of using them they might produce too little UV light to cure the enhancement. UV bulbs should be cured two to three times a year depending on its use. Choosing not to be changed regularly gives service breakdown, skin irritation, and product sensitivity due to inadequate cured gels.

Remember that UV gels can generate a lot of heat when used. The heat can be controlled by slowly inserting your hand into the UV lamp. This slows the gel reaction and generates less heat. The heat released is called an exothermic reaction for the gel that occurs as each chemical bond of the polymer is formed. The more chemical bonds that are formed when the gel cures, the more heat will be generated. In fact, the more chemical bonds created when the gel polymerizes, the stronger the gel becomes. Know that gel polishes do not dry; instead, they cure the product. Gel polishes usually do not thicken over time. In some gel polishes, the solvent does not evaporate.

In order to remove gel polish, nail technicians file the polish off using an abrasive or an electric file. Some gel polishes can be removed by soaking the nails in a solution of acetone for about five to ten minutes to soften them and allow the nail technicians to scrape them off with a wooden stick. Make sure you do not damage the natural plate. A damaged nail could lead to problems such as infection or cracking due to the decreased strength of the fingernail. Some professionals who provide enhancement services would ask the client if they would like to have the enhancement removed easily. If the client chooses to, then the nail technician would use a soak-off UV or LED gel as a base coat, and then perform the remainder of the service. A date will be arranged to have the client get her gels removed.

Keep in mind that UV and LED gels require maintenance on a regular basis and which also depends on how fast the nails grow. Maintenance can be carried out using a medium-abrasive file 180 grit to thin and shape the enhancement. Always be sure to follow the manufacturer's instructions. Before the nail gets filed, you need to clean the nail with the manufacturer's cleaner or isopropanol which removes oils from the fingernail and which gives better adhesion of the gel to the nail plate. Filing should be carried out with a lighter touch. Two methods for removing gels include hard UV gels which cannot be removed with acetone, and the other method involves soft UV gels which can be removed with acetone. When removing the inhibition layer from the UV gel, make sure you avoid cleaning the nail that puts the gel on the surface of the skin. Use a nail wipe and start at the top of the fingernail that is nearest the cuticle and wipe away from the cuticle to a free edge of the fingernail.

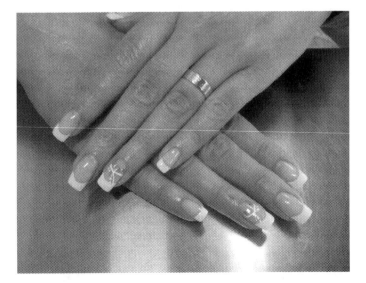

Chapter 5

Nail Products

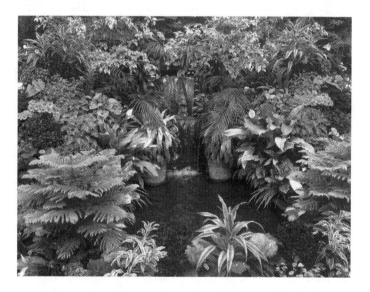

Chemical knowledge is important when using nail products. Your success depends on an understanding of chemicals and chemistry. You should not think that all chemicals are dangerous or harmful substances, but are helpful and beneficial to make your natural nails become beautiful. Everything around us are made of chemicals including the salon, the different types of cosmetics, vitamins, and even the water we drink and the gases of the atmosphere. Everything that we can see and touch except light and electricity is made of chemicals. The majority of chemicals are made of molecules which are considered to be tiny building blocks. They have the ability to be arranged and rearranged into different number of combinations. Remarkably, petroleum oil can actually be converted to Vitamin C, and even acetone can be converted to water and oxygen. There are so many possibilities.

A lot of us can distinguish between a solid and a liquid, but most people still have a difficult time distinguishing a vapor and a gas. Vapors form when liquids evaporate into the air. A liquid that is a liquid at room temperature can form a vapor. As the temperature increases, the faster a vapor will form. In fact, a vapor can turn back into a liquid if it is cooled again. The chemicals water, alcohol, and acetone have the ability to form vapors. Moreover, all types of nail enhancements form vapors as well as monomer liquids including odorless monomers, Ultraviolet gels, wrap resins and adhesives form vapors. They form vapors but not gases or fumes. Nail monomers give off vapors.

Let us now turn our attention to the terms adhesion, adhesives, and primers. Adhesion is a force that makes two surfaces to stick together. It takes place when molecules on one surface become attracted to molecules on another surface. Oils and waxes contaminates a surface and blocks adhesion. Clean dry surfaces provide better adhesion. Adhesives are chemicals that cause two surfaces to stick together. They allow incompatible surfaces to join together.

Nail primers are substances that improves adhesion. Nail polish base coats are a type of primer because the base coat makes the nail polish adhere better. Base coats act as an anchor and improves adhesion. There are other types of primers that are required with nail enhancements. There are three basic types which include acid-based, nonacid, and acid-free. This is important if you have oily nail plates where adhesion can be a problem and may lead to short and long term heath problems.

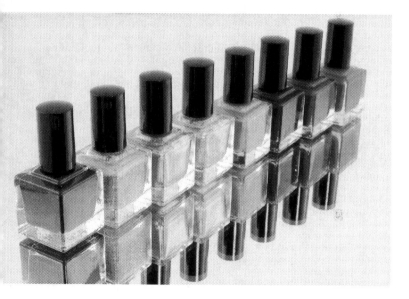

In fact, there are some nail primers that act as double-sided "sticky tape". One side of the primer sticks to the nail enhancement and the other side holds tightly onto the nail plate where they form physical bonds. New types of primers chemically bond with both the enhancement and the nail plate to create a chemical linkage. Do not think that nail primers etch the nail because they do not do so.

Nail clippings can actually soak for a long time in any primer without dissolving, but they still must be used with caution since some of them can be corrosive to soft tissues and the eyes. A corrosive is a substance that causes irreversible permanent skin or eye damage. Nail primers must never touch any part of the skin. Acid-base primers are corrosive and cause painful burns and scars to soft tissues and eyes. Corrosive primers should be kept in containers with child-resistant caps. Safety glasses should be worn when these products are used.

Although primers won't damage the nail plate, corrosive acid-based primers can actually burn the nail bed tissue if the nail plate is not properly filled. If you overfill the natural nail, it will excessively thin the nail and make it more porous. If too much primer is used, the nail plate can become overly saturated and tiny amounts might reach the nail bed which will then lead to the separation of the nail plate from the bed. The key point here is to use the primer sparingly. You only really need one very thin coat to put on your finger or toenail. If you are relying on two or more coats to prevent any lifting, then you know something is not right.

You will need to check your nail preparation and application procedures if there are any problems. Primers can become a crutch which covers up improper application or inadequate nail plate preparations. It is better to find out what the problem is and improve your technique using nail primer rather than relying on excessive amounts of primer.

Understand not all primers are corrosive to the skin. Noncorrosive primers are also called nonacid or acid-free primers that do not contain the chemical methacrylate which is the acid-base primer ingredient. Nonacid primers contain other kinds of acidic substances, whereas acid-free primers contain no acids and where the pH is neutral. Both types are noncorrosive to the skin and prevents burning of the soft tissue.

They need to be used with caution and skin contact should be avoided. Repeated skin contact caused by an improper application leads to allergic reactions over time. Without using the product, it is not likely you will become allergic to the product. Vapors formed as products don't cause skin allergies. Allergies are caused by repeated products applied to the skin. Furthermore, it is best to avoid contact between nail enhancement products and soft tissues.

Remember that good adhesion depends on proper technique and using the best and highly-quality products. Always start with a clean and dry surface. Always wash your hands and feet and scrub the nail plate to remove surface oils and contaminants that interfere with proper adhesion procedures. Scrubbing also gets rid of bacteria and fungi which cause nail infections. It is not a good idea to skip this step because it can lead to product lifting at the base of the nail plate near the eponychium. Not preparing properly for this procedure can produce nail enhancement product lifting.

Nail dehydrators removes surface moisture from the nail plate. A lot of moisture on the surface of the plate interferes with product adhesion just as much as surface oils can. Nail dehydrators have the ability to remove traces of moisture and oil. It only takes about 30 minutes for normal natural oils and moisture to return to the nail plate. Dehydrate only one hand or foot at a time and after thorough scrubbing for best results.

Roughing up your nails is harmful and should not be done. Adhesion works best when the nail plate is clean and dry. It is best to use a medium fine (240 grit) abrasive or buffer to remove just the surface shine. It is not a good idea to use heavy-grit abrasives, heavy-handed filing, and improper use of electric files since these strip away the layer of the natural nail plate. Remember the thinner the nail plate, the weaker it tends to be. Thinner nail plates create weaker foundations for nail enhancements. You want the nail plate to be thicker to serve as a better foundation. You will have better success wearing nail enhancements if you don't overfile the nail plate. Again, you want to keep the nail plate thick, strong, and healthy.

Do not mistaken that primers and nail enhancements cause the problems for nail damage. Rough filing damages the nail plate and underlying sensitive tissues of the nail bed. Heavy abrasives and overfiling, which is excessively roughing up the nail plate, can cause the nail plate to lift and separate from the nail bed. Overfiling causes dangerous and excessive thinning of the nail plate. If this happens, you are susceptible to developing infections under the nail plate.

In fact, overfiling the nail plate cause nail enhancement use to be useless. It leads to lifting, breaking, free-edge chipping, and free-edge product separation or "curling". It also promotes allergic reactions and cause painful friction burns to soft tissues of the nail bed. It is better to remove all dead tissue from the side walls and cuticle area, and above all removing bacteria, fungi, oil, and moisture from the nail plate. Improper nail preparation leads to problems.

Soaking the nail plate in a liquid including water or acetone will temporarily soften the nail plate's surface for about an hour. Using metal or wooden pushers to scrape residual products leads to pitting and gouging the nail surface. Avoid heavy-handed scraping and filing to protect your nails from excessive damage. If the coating is not all removed after exposing it to remover solvents, more time should be allowed for the remover to soften the coating so then it can be gently removed without damage.

A lot of ladies like to apply coatings to the nail plate. Coatings are products that cover the nail plate where the film is hardened. Coatings include nail polish, top coats, nail enhancements, and adhesives. There are two main types of coatings which include coating that polymerize or cure which is a type of chemical reaction and coatings that harden upon evaporation which is a type of physical reaction. Nail enhancements and Ultraviolet Gel manicures are coatings created by chemical reactions, whereas nail polish, base and top coats are examples of coatings formed by evaporation.

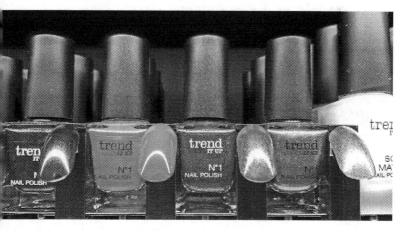

Let us take a closer look at the chemistry of these products. Nail enhancements are chemical reactions. Over a trillion molecules react to make one sculptered nail. Both durable and long lasting coatings or nail enhancements are made by chemical reactions. With that being said, monomer liquid and polymer powder nail enhancements, Ultraviolet gels, wraps, and adhesives are more examples of chemical reactions.

The molecules in the final product join together in very long chains with each chain containing millions of molecules. The gigantic chains of molecules are called polymers which can be liquid but are usually solid. Chemical reactions that make polymers are called polymerization. In the nail industry, they use the terms cure, curing, or hardening. It is worth noting that there are many different types of polymers. Nylon and hair are examples of polymers as well as proteins being polymers. Nail plates are made up of proteins which include keratin. Nail plates and hair made from polymers. Individual molecules join to make the polymer are called monomers that make up polymers. Amino Acids are considered to be monomers that join together to make a polymer called keratin.

Understanding polymerization is critical to prevent problems involving nails. Monomer liquid, polymer powder nail enhancements, and ultraviolet gels and wraps might seem different, but are in fact similar. Each of the products is made from different but closely related monomers. An initiator is a chemical ingredient that triggers polymerization. Initiator molecules have energy. Each time an initiator reacts with a monomer, the initiator excites it with a boost of energy, but the monomers don't like the extra energy and want to get rid of it. They attach themselves to the tail end of another monomer and continue to pass the energy along, and then the second monomer does it best to get rid of the energy. The chain of monomers get longer and longer. Billions of monomers attach each other in less than a second. Many of the growing monomer chains become entangled and knotted which explains why the product begins to thicken. The chains become too long and crowded to move around freely. The product becomes a mass of micrscopic-sized strings where the surface becomes hard to file. It takes several days before the chains reach their full length. Thus, we can state that nail enhancements become stronger during the first 48 hours. Initiators get extra energy they pass on from either heat or light. Liquid and powder systems have the ability to use thermal initiators. They gather energy from the heat waves of the room or from the heat waves of the hand. Ultraviolet curing products use photoinitiators and derive their extra energy when exposed to ultraviolet light.

Catalysts are substances that speed up a chemical reaction but they do not get consumed. They make initiators work more efficiently and by carrying out chemical reactions more smoother. Catalysts are found in many nail enhancement products and explains why nail enhancements harden very quickly.

Oligomers are short chain of monomers that have stopped growing into polymers. They are useful because they can be joined quickly into long chains to create polymers. They are ingredients in ultraviolet gels and give the gels their sticky consistency. If were not oligomers, ultraviolet gel products can take two to three hours to harden into nail enhancements instead of a few minutes.

There are simple and cross-linking of polymer chains. The head of one monomer has the ability to react with the tail of another monomer and the process continues. The final result is a long chain of monomers attached from head to tail. We call these simple polymer chains. Examples of simple polymer chains includes wraps and tip adhesives. The tangled chains are unraveled by solvents and explains why they are removed. Polymer chains can also be unraveled by force. Products involving these simple polymer chains can be damaged by sharp impacts or even by heavy stresses. Molecules such as dyes and stains can also be mixed with these tangled chains. Nail polish, marker ink, and food cause unsightly stains on the surface.

There has to be a way to overcome these problems. Ultraviolet Gels and monomer liquid and polymer powder nail enhancements use a special type of small amounts of monomers called cross-linkers. Cross-linkers are monomers that joins different polymer chains together. It is these cross-links that create strong net-like polymers. The three-dimensional structure has great strength and flexibility which we call a nail enhancement.

Nail plates and hair also have cross-links which makes them tough and durable. They increase the strength of the natural nails and nail enhancements, and the cross links makes them more resistant to staining. On the other hand, cross-links are resistant to solvent such as water and acetone because cross-link enhancements take longer to remove in acetone than products that are not cross-linked such as wraps and tip adhesives, and this explains why they are more more resistant to water.

All nail enhancements and adhesives fall in the category of chemical ingredients called acrylics. There are three types of acrylics used to make nail enhancements such as methacrylates, acrylates, and cyanoacrylates. Methacrylates are considered to be used to make all monomer liquid and polymer powder systems and ultraviolet gel. Other ultraviolet gels are based on another type of acrylic called acrylates. All nail adhesives and wraps are based on cyanoacrylates. The physical and chemical properties of these different types of acrylates makes their chemistry unique. Yet, the chemistry involving nail enhancement products and adhesives are similar.

Methyl methacrylate monomer is abbreviated as MMA, and it is a chemical that has both positive and negative effects. MMA is used for bone repair cement for implantation into the body, does not get absorbed into the blood to affect health, and does not cause brain tumors. However, MMA is a poor ingredient for nail enhancements and should not be used. MMA nail products don't adhere well to the nail plate without roughing up the surface of the nail plate using an abrasive or electric file. Too much thinning of the nail plate makes it weaker. Another disadvantage using MMA is that it creates nails that are rigid and difficult to break. If MMA is jammed, the overly filled or thinned natural nail plate will break and cause serious nail damage.

MMA is difficult to remove and does not dissolve in product removers. It gets pried off and creates more damage, and above all MMA products have the ability to discolor and become brittle more quickly than traditional products and must be removed more often. This is terrible since it is difficult to remove it and causes a lot of nail damage.

So now you have a better understanding

of polymerization. Let us take a look at evaporation coatings. Nail polishes, top coats, and base coats can also form coatings, but the products are entirely different. They don't polymerize or cure. There are no chemical reactions, and they contain no monomers or oligomers. The products work by evaporation only. Most of the ingredients are volatile which means they evaporate quickly. More specifically, we are talking about the solvents evaporating quickly. There are special polymers that are dissolved in these solvents, and these polymers are not considered to be cross-linked polymers which makes them dissolve more easily. As the solvent evaporates, the polymer gives a smooth film. The film can hold pigments which gives its color. The types of products formed contain ingredients called plasticizers which are used to keep the products flexible and ultraviolet stabilizers which also control color stability and prevent sunlight from causing fading or discoloration. It is these ingredients that are found in nail enhancement products. Remember that the strength of non-crosslinked polymers is lower than cross-linked nail enhancement polymers. This explains why polishes are more likely to be prone to chipping and dissolve more readily by removers. I hope this explains the different between coatings that polymerize and those that have the ability to harden upon evaporation. Remember all nail enhancements are made from organic chemicals.

The human nail is made up of the nail plate, nail matrix, nail folds, nail bed, cuticle, and hyponchium. Human nails are made up of hard keratin which contains more sulfur than normal skin keratin. The hardness of nails depends on the number of keratin fibers and disulfide bonds connecting cysteine components of keratin together. Nails also contain water, lipids, and small amounts of calcium, iron, aluminum, copper, zinc, and other metals. Normal water content of human nails is in the range of 10% - 15% with an average of 12%. Lipids are present in a small amount which is about 5%. Lipids contribute to the flexibility of nails. Since there is a low concentration of lipids, the nail plate is 1000-fold more permeable to water than skin. This is why nails can be hydrated and dehydrated for proper hand and foot care.

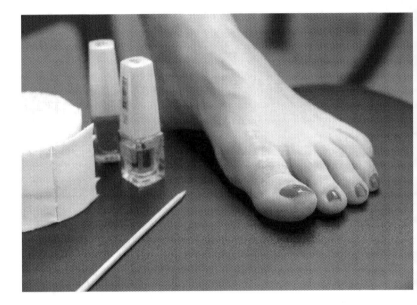

Average fingernail growth is about 0.1 mm per day or 3 mm per month. Fingernails have the ability to grow out completely in 6 months. Toenails grow out at 1/3 to 1/2 rate of fingernails and take 12 - 18 months to grow out completely. Nail growth is greatly influenced by weather. They grow slower at night and during winter. Different nail care products include hardeners which are designed to protect the layer on the nail plate. They increase the hardness and strength of the nail and have a chemical cross-linking agent. The composition is similar to ordinary clear nail polish. They are considered to be functional nail care products. Nail moisturizers increase the hardness of nails by containing moisturizing ingredients. They include lotions or creams applied to the nail plate. Nail polish consist of pigments which are suspended in a volatile non-aqueous solvent and in which film-formers are added. Adding pearlescent and metallic ingredients and shimmers provide great effects. Cuticle removers remove the cuticle and are formulated as liquid or cream and contain alkali ingredients to get rid of the cuticle keratin. Artificial nails contain preformed plastics, formed acrylics, and both. Formed acrylic gels are mixtures of acrylic monomers and polymers which has the tendency to harden on the nail's surface.

Nail polish removers are organic solvents to remove nail polish. Oils and fragrances can be added in the formulations. Nail care products can also affect human nails. Using detergents and overuse of nail polish removers damages the keratin and decreases water content that leads to brittleness. Moisturizers might help maintain nail hydration by sealing moisture that would evaporate.

Let us look at functional nail care products more closely. Functional nail care products maintain nail hardness. Nail hardeners harden brittle nails. They function as a base coat. Most nail hardeners contain a chemical cross-linking agent such as formalin and dimethyl urea. The ingredients react with keratin on the nail and create more cross-links which hardens the nail. However, too many links can cause the nails to become dry and brittle. Nail hardeners should only be applied to the free edge of the nails while shielding the skin.

Note that formalin is a 37% solution of formaldehyde in water. Formalin contains methylene glycol, water, small amounts of methanol, methylene glycols, and a small amount of formaldehyde. Formaldehyde has actually been replaced with polyesters, polyamides, and acrylate polymers. Substances more likely to be present in nail hardeners include toluene, nitrocellulose, acrylate polymers, resins, acetates, proteins, biotin, nylon, glycerin, propylene glycol, and salts of different metals. Products that don't contain cross-linking agents are referred to as "nonhardening" nail polish or base coat. They can also increase nail hardness due to resins and polymers.

Nail moisturizers add moisture to the nail plate. They contain moisturizing ingredients such as occlusives, emollients, humectants, and proteins. Ingredients that increase water-binding capacity include urea and lactic acid. Nail moisturizers should be applied under cotton gloves and during night times. Cuticles remover dissolve excess cuticular tissue on the nail plate by attacking disulfide bonds of cysteine in keratin. They are water-based formulations. They are available as liquids, gels, or creams and contain cuticle-dissolving agents such as sodium hydroxide and potassium hydroxide. They have a highly alkaline pH and is irritating to the skin. Milder preparations contain trisodium phosphate or tetrasodium pyrophosphate. Ingredients such as water, emollients, humectants, thickners, and preservatives are added to these formulations. There are even cuticle softeners which only wear down the cuticle for mechanical removal by subsequent trimming. They contain quartenary ammonium compounds in a very low concentration.

As discussed earlier, nail polish contain base coats, top coats, and nail polish. Ingredients include resins, solvents, plasticizers, color additives, thixotropic agents, color stabilizers/UV absorbents. Let us take the time to review the major ingredients of nail polish again. Base coats are clear solutions that are applied to the clean nail plate. They enhance healthy growth of nails and contain nutrients and moisturizers. They also make sure the nail polish does not stain the nails. They also create a smooth nail surface which the nail lacquer has better adhesion. They also contain more secondary film-formers than primary film-formers and are also less viscous than colored nail polish.

Top coats are clear solutions that are applied over nail polish. They add a protective layer and prevent the applied nail polish from fading and chipping. They also enhance gloss and reduce drying time. They also have an increased amount of primary film-formers, more plasticizers, and less secondary film-formers. They are also less viscous than color nail polish. Nail polish is a colored suspension that contain volatile solvents and contain viscosity modifying agents. Nail polish contain a lot of different ingredients that can be categorized into basic groups. Raw materials applied to base coats, top coats, and nail polish are about the same, but the percentage of ingredients is different. Resins are also known as film-formers that hold ingredients of the lacquer together and in which forms a strong film on the nails. Resins are also polymers that are solid of soft solid in a pure state. The help improve adhesion of the product to the nail. They also have the ability to give the polish a glossy appearance. There are two types of resins known as hard, glossy resins which are called primary film-formers and soft, pliable resins which are known as secondary film-formers. Both of them are used in different concentrations that depend on the desired effect of the nail polish.

Hard, glossy resins give the lacquered nail a hard, brittle film. These type of resins include nitrocellulose, vinyl polymers, methacrylate, and acrylate polymers or copolymers, acrylate esters, acrylamide, as well as derivatives of cellulose such as cellulose acetate proprionate. In fact, nitrocellulose is a primary film-forming agent in nail polish. This type of film is oxygen permeable allowing the exchange of gases between the atmosphere and nail plate. Softer more pliable resins enhance adhesion and give gloss, flexibility, and resistance performance. Examples of these kind of resins include toluene sulfonamide/ epoxy resin, polyester resins, acrylate, and metaacrylate copolymers, and polyvinyl butyral. Base coats have a higher proportion of pliable resins. Proper ratios of the two types of film formers are needed to provide formulations to obtain films that have drying time and are flexible.

Solvents dissolve resins, pigments, and evaporate that leaves a smooth film. They also have regular viscosity, application, flow, leveling, drying time, hardness, gloss, and give stability. Blending solvents give an optimal level of physical and chemical properties. Examples of solvents used in nail polish formulations include alkyl esters such as ethyl acetate and n-butyl acetate, glycol ethers such as propylene glycol monomethyl ether, alcohols such as isopropyl alcohol and alkanes such as hexane and heptane.

Plasticizers improve resin flexibility and also chip resistance. Used plasticizers include camphor, castor oil, glyceral tribenzoate, glycerol, triphenyl phosphate, trimethyl pentamyl diisobutyrate, acetyl tributyl citrate, ethyl tosylamide, sucrose benzoate, ethyl toluene sulfonamide, and polymer plasticizers called NEPLAST which is a polyether-urethane.

Color additives give a variety of shades. They should be insoluble in solvents in order to avoid staining and discoloration of nails and to avoid chemical reactions to the lacquer. Lakes are most often used for nail polish. A shimmer effect gets created by incorporating powdered aluminum, mica flakes, and bismuth oxychloride. Thixotropic agents are also known as thickeners or suspending agents. They provide flow control and keep color additives dispersed. They increase nail polish viscosity and become fluid when shaking the bottle or brushing. Base coats and top coats are uncolored formulations and do not require thickeners since they don't contain suspended particles. Clay derivatives such as stearalkonium bentonite or stearalkonium hectorite can be used. Silica is also used as a thickener.

Color stabilizers or UV absorbents prevent color shifting of nail polish due to exposure to UV light. Some top coats contain UV filters that prevent fading over time. Examples of color stabilizers include benzophenone-1 and etocrylene. UV filters that are found in nail polish formulations and top coats provide color protection. They are also nail treatment ingredients which include compounds that strengthen the nails and enhance nail health. Examples of these ingredients include vitamins, minerals, vegetable oils, herbal extracts, and fibers such as silk and poly-ureaurethane. Poly-ureaurethane manages signs and symptoms of nail dystrophy such as nail splitting and nail fragility. Tolnaftate can be used an an antifungal agent incorporated in nail polish formulations that takes care of fungal infection of the nails.

Let us take a look at additional types of nail polish. Water-based nail polish seems promising. Although evaporating water is slow, they are still inexpensive, nonflammable, and odorless. Adding preservatives can even prevent microbial growth over time. Magnetic nail polish contains iron powder. There is a tiny magent built into the cap of the nail polish container. It is held over the nail before solvents evaporate which causes the iron powder in the formulation to gravitate toward the magent and form a pattern. Photocured is also known as UV-cured nail polish or shellac nail polish. They contain the same pigments as nail polish formulations, but instead of using a solvent/resin base they have methacrylate or acrylate oligomers and monomers. They also have a photoinitiator which causes polymerization when exposed to UV light and which also leaves a polymer/

pigment coat. Photocured products provide a thin coat that is harder, shinier, longer lasting, and more resistant to chipping. UV curing usually take about ten minutes.

Let us take a look at how nail polish is formulated. Colored nail polish are made as suspensions. The process consist of formulating the pigment blend, formulating the nail polish base, and coloring the laquer base. Pigment preparation is a critical step. The finer the pigment is grounded, the higher the gloss and more stable the product. Pigments are normally prepared in "chip form". They are mixed with nitrocellulose and plasticizer using a high-shear mixer. The resulting mixture gets passed through a mill and split into solid fragments.

Usually small-scale size preparations, pigments are prewetted by making a 1:1 or

1:2 premix in the carrier under slow stirring conditions. The polish base is prepared by blending the components with sufficient stirring. During the last step, color mixture is dispersed in the nail polish during stirring. Other solvents and additional ingredients are added to the mixture. The thixotropic agent gets added and the viscosity is adjusted.

Let us take a look now at artificial nails. We now know they are longer lasting than natural nails and highly resistant to cracking and chipping. Nail tips are made up of nylon or plastic. They are either preglued or they must be glued before applying them. The glue is considered to be an adhesive which is methacrylate-based or cyanoacrylate-based glue. They are normally placed on the nail plate for about five to ten seconds for proper adhesion. Tips can also be reshaped and colored.

Sculptured nails are known as acrylic nails and porcelain nails. Building custom-made nails are sculpted on a template that is attached to the natural nail plate. Basic steps include cleansing and filing, putting the sculpture form, primary, mixing, sculpting, and finishing the process. A solvent such as isopropyl alcohol is applied to the nail plate in order to remove nail polish residue and oils. The nails' surface is abraded with a pumice stone or it can be filed further to clean the nail plate and create an optimal surface for adhesion of the sculpted nail. A flexible template such as Teflon is placed under the natural nail plate. The procedure provides additional surface for the natural nail plate. Primers are also applied to the nail plate before sculpting. Primers are substances that help with adhesion. Most of the primers act as a double-sided tape where one side sticks to the nail enhancement and the other side holds onto the nail plate.

Sculpturing is performed by applying layers of acrylic polymers on the natural nails' surface and template using a brush. The brush is dipped into a liquid monomer and drawn through a polymer powder. A small bead forms at the end of the brush. Once sculpturing is done, the hardened polymers get shaped into the desried length and width. The template can be removed from the fingers. Note that monomer liquids are made up of ethyl methacrylate and other methacrylate monomers that provide cross-linking inhibitors such as hydroquinone that slows down polymerization, UV stabilizers, catalysts, flexibilizing agents, and other additives. The powder polymer consists of methyl and/or ethyl methacrylate polymer coated with benzoyl peroxide that acts as a polymerization initiator.

The final stage of the nail sculpture gets sanded to a high shine. Nail polish, decals, and decorative arrangements can be added. The nails harden at room temperature because a chemical reaction between the liquid and the powder polymer. Artificial nails are not designed to be taken off on a frequent basis. Sometimes, when the process is done carefully, completely removing them can damage and dry the nail plate.

The are variations of the sculpturing technique. Plastic tips can be used for sculpturing nails. The tips are glued only to the tip of the nails. The nail plate itself is filled with acrylic polymers such as liquid and powder. Applying tips reduces the sculpturing time. Some artificial nails cure under UV light; thus they are called UV gels. As discussed earlier in this book, UV gels do not cure at room temperature. Nails are placed under a UV lamp for a few minutes. They are considered a one-phase system which includes polymerization photoinitiators, urethane methacrylate oligomers, cross-linking monomers, and catalysts.

Nail polish removers take off the lacquer by redissolving the resins. Ingredients include organic solvents such as acetone. Some nail polish removers contain emollients to conter dehydration and brittleness effects of these solvents and help condition the skin. Fragrances, color additives, and preservatives might be added to make the nail polish remover more friendly.

Solutions, cleaning pads, and sponges are types of nail polish removers. Solutions can be applied with either a cotton ball or tissue and wiped over the nail to remove the fingernail polish. Cleaning pads are pads that are prewetted with a nail polish remover solution. A piece of foam sponge gets soaked with the solution in a container with a hole at its center. Fingers are dipped into the sponge through the hole so the polish can be removed.

Typical quality problems in nail care products include bubbling, cracking, chipping, and thickening. Bubbling happens during application. It is caused by air that may come from "over-shaked" bottles. Oil residue can also cause bubbling or perhaps the thickening of the product. When they get applied, the microstructure collapses and solvents cannot escape during drying and remain captured in the final film. Note that bubbles lead to chipping when dry.

Cracking has to do with the nail polish film being uneven, and there is cracking on the surface. The flexibility of the film might be inappropriate which results from a abnormally low plasticizer concentration. Remember that plasticizers make the film formed on the nails more flexible which decreases rigidity. If the concentration is too low, a rigid film develops which can not adjust itself to the nails natural curvature. "Cracked" or "crackel" nail polish shatters as it does and gives a artistic chipped effect. Crackle nail polish forces the layer to separate into randomly placed cracks. Ethanol is added to the formulation that causes quick drying after application.

Chipping has to do with small, broken, or missing nail polish film pieces from the nail plates. Normally, it happens after a few days wearing at the tip of the nail plates. The source of the problem has to do with poor flexibility of the nail polish film. It could also happen if there are too many layers or too thick layers are applied that makes the final film rigid. Plasticizers which have appropriate concentrations prevents this phenomenon. Thickening has to do with the viscosity of a product being increase compared to the starting viscosity. Correct consistencies help with the application of at least one coat of enamel before the brush is redipped. The efficiency of diluent solvents normally decreases over time that may cause the thickening of the product. Part of the volatile solvents can evaporate and cause thickening.

Let us take the time to evaluate nail care products. Parameters include abrasion resistance, gloss, film flexibility, and hardness, drying time, adhesion test, brushability, color, dispersion of pigments, and viscosity. Manufacturers determine the range of acceptance and other limiting factors. Let us first talk about abrasion resistance. Nail polish films come into contact with many objects being worn. Abrasion resistance of the film determines the longevity of films on the nails. The "abraser" is a machine that consists of two abrasive wheels that produce rub-wear action. During the process, nail polish is applied to the steel panel. The wheels rotate while sliding on the sample film which also forms a characteristic pattern on the film. This could be interpreted as a decrease in film thickeners after a certain number of cycles. This is referred to as depth of wear. Weight loss after a number of cycles is also another interpretation. This is also referred to as the wear index. Another possible interpretation could be the number of abrasion cycles required to wear through the coating of known thickness.

Let us talk about gloss. Gloss is an optical property on a surface such as a nail polish film that is characterized by the ability to reflect light. Gloss can be measured by shining light at a surface and determining the amount of light reflected. A glossmeter is a machine that directs light at a specific angle to test surface and at the same time measure the amount of reflection. Intensity depends on the material and angle of illumination. A lot of industries have adopted the 20/60/85 degrees geometries which refers to the angle of incident light. The measurements are then compared to the amount of reflected light from a black, highly polished gloss standard with a defined refractive index. The standard's reflectance is 100 gloss units (GUs). The scale is suitable for non-metallic films such as plastics and paints that fall within this range. Note that the number is not a value in percentage. Materials such as mirrors have higher refractive index than nail polish and the black standard. Higher values of 100 can be found. By using a glossmeter, differences in gloss invisible to human eyes can be measured.

Let us take a look at film flexibility and hardness. Scratch testing is another method that is used to characterize surface mechanical properties of thin films and coatings. The process of scratching can be done by pencils or other tools with sharp tips. Scratch hardners can be measured by moving a sharp object under a known pressure over a test surface. The results can be either the value of the load pressure to scratch through the test material if a scratching tool of constant hardness is used, or the hardness of the scratching tool becomes varied while keeping the load pressure constant.

Let us take a look at drying time. Application, performance, and drying time depend on volatility of solvents. If the drying process is too fast, there won't be enough time to spread and level the film on the nails. If the drying process is slow, the film won't set on the nails and can be transferred to surfaces the customer touches. Drying time is measured on a clean glass/metal surface by applying a thin film coating and measuring the time for complete drying of the film.

Let us take a look at the Adhesion Test. To make sure the nail polish coatings perform satisfactorily, they need to adhere to the nails. Many methods can be used to determine how well a nail polish coating bonds to the nail plate. Measuring techniques such as using a tape, a knife, or a pull-off adhesion tester can be used. When using the tape test, a pressure-sensitive tape is put on diagonally across a coated surface. A specific cut pattern is formed on its surface. After applying tape, it is pulled back slowly. Any amount of coating removed from the surface has to do with the adhesives of the nail polish to the nail or primer. When using the knife test, a knife is used to remove the film from the surface. The pull-off test is more quantitative. A loading fixture, or a dolly, is affixed by an adhesive to a coating. Loads are applied to the surface until the dolly is pulled off. The force required to pull off the dolly off or the force the dolly withstands gives the tensile strength. The other test worth mentioning is the Brushability Test. When applying nail polish to nails, ladies want the product to provide a smooth film without streaking. Lower-viscosity nail polish allows an even application and better spreading of the nail polish. Thin films are formed and more than two layers are needed to achieve the desired color. Higher viscosity transfers more of the product to the nail plates. Brushing can result in streaks and drying time can be lengthened. Brushability can be tested by applying the product to a test surface and by checking the smoothness of the surface.

There are ingredients that can cause safety concerns. Nail care formulations have flammable ingredients. They should not be kept close to a heat source. Toluene, phthalates, and methylene glycol are safety concerns. Symptoms include irritation to the eyes and nose, headache, dizziness, and drowsiness. Toluene is a solvent in nail polish, nail hardeners, and even nail polish removers. Phthalates are used in nail care products as plasticizers to make nail polish films flexible and resistant against chipping.

These ingredients are used in cosmetics, plastics, and toys. Methylene glycol or formaldehyde is an ingredient found in nail hardeners. It alters the structure of the nail plate by cross-linking the keratin. Formaldehyde, however, causes nail brittleness, irritation, or allergic reactions for those who are sensitive to it. It can lead to cancer through inhalation. Methylene glycol is nonvolatile so it is not present in high concentration in the air. Formaldehyde and methylene glycol can be considered to be safe when used at a maximal effective concentration. The formalin concentration should not exceed 0.2% by weight. However, both formaldehyde and methylene glycol can be safe in nail care products based on research studies.

Finally, packing of nail care products

include glass bottles, plastic bottles, soft tubes, and pastic jar. Nail polish and nail hardeners are kept in glass bottles with different shapes. Even liquid cuticle removers cab be packaged into glass bottles. Some applicator brish is attached to the cap of the bottle, and there are some nail polish removers that are packages into glass bottles. Nail polish removers are also packaged in simple plastic bottles. Cuticle softener, cuticle remover, and nail moisturizer products are available on soft tubes that are fitted with a nozzle applicator. Nail polish removers that have a piece of sponge soaked with a nail polish remover solution are supplied in jars. A hole is found in the middle of the sponges where consumers dip their fingers into the sponge through the hole. Nail polish remover pads get prewetted with a nail polish remover solution and are supplied in plastic jars. Some manufacturers package these pads individually. Even nail moisturizers can be packaged into plastic jars. As for nail tips, they are available to use already and can be supplied in a kit with the necessary tools and ingredients.

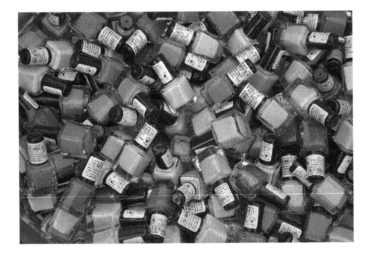

Final Thoughts

Your nails can either make you look beautiful or not look good at all. Your hands and feet speak for you. Meeting ladies dressed in a professional manner and are well-groomed is more pleasing than meeting ladies whose appearance seems repulsive. A great deal of chemistry is involved when it comes to the nail industry and their products such as manicuring, pedicuring, electric filing, nail tips and wraps, monomer liquid and polymer powder nail enhancements, UV and LED Gels, and even making that creative artistic touch on your nails. As the fields of science and technology changes so will the cosmetics industry. The future of nails can change and will get better. Creative innovations of new products that will help keep the nails healthy and looking beautiful will be even more impressive and may help us live longer and happy lives!

References

Voet, Donald and Voet, Judith G. Biochemistry Second Edition. John Wiley & Sons, Inc. 1995

Zumdahl, Steven S. and Zumdahl, Susan A. Chemistry Sixth Edition. Houghton Mifflon Company. 2003

Timberlake, Karen C. Ninth Edition. Benjamin Cummings. 2006

Botero, Alisha Rimando, Halal, John, Kilgore, Mary Ann, Mcconnell, Jim, Mccormick, Janet, Peters, Vicki, Schoon, Douglas, Spear, Jeryl Milady Nail Technology Seventh Edition. Cengage Learning. 2015

Baki, Gabriella and Alexander, Kenneth S. Introduction to Cosmetic Formulation and Technology. John Wiley & Sons. 2015

https://pixabay.com/photos/
azalea-waterfall-garden-pond-water-5120368/

https://pixabay.com/illustrations/
science-periodic-table-elements-2227606/

https://pixabay.com/photos/
laboratory-chemistry-science-glass-4415978/

https://pixabay.com/photos/
laboratory-chemistry-chemical-1009178/

https://pixabay.com/photos/
clamy-nail-polish-mirror-nail-polish-4331963/

https://pixabay.com/photos/
stream-waterfall-zen-landscape-970568/

https://pixabay.com/photos/
color-nails-tips-honeycomb-3239832/

https://pixabay.com/photos/
summer-sea-varnish-sand-seashells-1363056/

https://pixabay.com/photos/
hands-manicure-female-nails-hand-4190681/

https://pixabay.com/photos/
cosmetology-polishing-red-beauty-1471324/

https://pixabay.com/photos/
waterfall-garden-nature-tropical-1037048/

https://pixabay.com/photos/
fingernails-hands-nail-design-259972/

https://pixabay.com/photos/
water-summer-sea-nail-polish-3247286/

https://pixabay.com/photos/
nail-polish-nail-varnish-fingernails-281878/

https://pixabay.com/illustrations/
fingernail-salon-nails-manicure-5316581/

https://pixabay.com/photos/
waterfall-chinese-garden-australia-465089/

https://pixabay.com/photos/
nail-gel-beauty-manicure-nails-gel-5186206/

https://pixabay.com/photos/
gel-manicure-brush-template-hand-2253782/

https://pixabay.com/photos/
nail-varnish-nail-gel-fingernails-2112366/

https://pixabay.com/photos/nail-gel-manicure-657597/

https://pixabay.com/photos/
garden-water-landscape-flowers-944438/

https://pixabay.com/photos/
nailvarnish-cosmetics-trend-series-3905479/

https://pixabay.com/photos/
manicure-pedicure-cosmetics-870857/

https://pixabay.com/photos/
foot-foot-care-ten-barefoot-skin-2488529/

https://pixabay.com/photos/
varnish-varnishes-paint-toenail-418241/

About the Author

Harminder Gill finished his undergraduate studies at the University of California, Riverside, where he finished his bachelor of science degree in biological chemistry with an emphasis in chemistry. After completing his undergraduate studies, he attended graduate school at the University of California, Davis, where he finished his master's degree in organic chemistry. After carrying out several teaching assignments, he went into the teaching profession at community colleges. He was an Adjunct Professor at many different community colleges, and he became a life member for both alumni associations at UCR and

UCD. He has done homeschooling and tutoring throughout many communities both in person and world-wide online where he offers several different academic subjects from the humanities, social sciences, physical sciences, life sciences, engineering sciences, and test preparation. Plently of his students have done and continue to do excetionally well, including those who have achieved high scores on standardized tests, getting accepted into training academies, universities, and programs of their choice. He has served on board of directors, completed the Distinguished Toastmaster (DTM) in the Toastmasters Program for Public Speaking and Leadership, and continues to do research in the cosmetics industry and keeps current in the math, sciences, and technology.

Printed in the United States
By Bookmasters